Maxine Taylor

Secrets

from the

Womb

The Hidden Pact that Runs Your Life

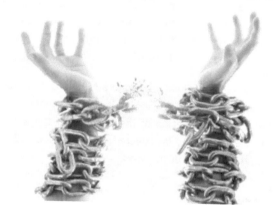

Produced by Starmax Astrology.

Published by Long Story Short Publishing Company

ISBN paperback: 978-1-960995-25-4

ISBN eBook: 978-1-960995-26-1

Photo by Shantell Cescutti

Contents

With Gratitude

To Denise Cassino, my dear friend and
publicist/publisher:
Thank you, Denise, for the answer.

Thank you

This book is dedicated to all the people
who gave me permission
to share their stories with you.
May they inspire and encourage you.

A Must-Read Message from Maxine

DEAR READER,

I am thrilled to be able to share the information in this book with you. It contains the answers to the questions I have asked for years. It represents the end of my story and the beginning of a new life.

Those of you who have followed me for any length of time know how passionate I am about helping people identify and release their childhood programming. Early on in my long astrological career, I realized that the birth chart contains this programming, but doesn't tell you how to release it. This led me to develop my Take Back Your Life method, which goes beyond astrology. Any topic can be plugged into TBYL: money, love, sex, health, career, etc. It is eye opening and, in many cases, life transforming. Because I also recognized the power and destructiveness of the Bad Message we received when we were very little, I began every session and every book I wrote with how to identify and release this message. But it never really left. I *had* to get to the source of its power. I *had* to find out why I and everyone else would continue to return to the Bad Message.

So, I asked God to give me the answer. And the next day, I shared my frustration with my dear friend and publicist/publisher, Denise Cassino, who delivered God's answer: "Go back to the womb." And as she described what it had meant to her to take this step with her psychotherapist, I consciously moved back into my mother's womb. It was as simple as that. No big deal. And the result was powerful! In a split second I saw my life in clear vision! Suddenly, my whole life made sense! All I could say to Denise was, "Wow!" I found myself in a state of love, joy and bliss that words cannot describe. I tingled all over my body. I was truly happy. Some call this state the present, the quantum field, the zero - point field, the unified field, oneness, source energy, the I Am, etc. I call it the magic. It is our natural state because love, joy, bliss, happiness, health, wealth – all the good stuff! – is who we are. The magic is your natural state. It is who you are and what you are.

I stayed in the magic for a few days, after which time I lost my love, joy and bliss. It felt like I was back at square one. Words cannot describe the conflict between the rarified air of the magic and the pain of being out of it. This was my clear signal it was time for the next step. I felt it. I knew it. So, once again, I asked God what that step was. Instantly, I got my answer: the Pact. Of course! That made perfect sense! It's the Pact with our mother that seals the deal.

My Pact with my mother was very clear to me, so I let it go to God. Once again, I instantly moved into the magic where, in addition to experiencing love, joy and bliss, I felt liberated, energized and free to do what I wanted. I was empowered!

True to form, though, a few days later, I lost my love, joy and bliss. I knew it was time to deal with the Bad Message and its power.

In my Take Back Your Life books and sessions I began with the Bad Message and from there, moved on to the commitment to our mother. The commitment to her is *strong*; the Pact with her is *powerful!* This explains why releasing the Bad Message was not enough – it wasn't the first step! The Pact was!

Even though I had dealt with the Bad Message for years, I went through it again, but this time I was able to see it clearly, through the eyes of truth. As I replayed it mentally, I stopped at the critical point – the point that showed me I was not bad! I was actually good! I had *not* broken my pact with my mother – it was *she* who had not taken her responsibility with *me*! I had never seen this before! I released the scene in which I bought the lie that I was bad, and accepted the truth that I was good. I kept repeating to myself, "I am good! I am good!" For the first time in my life, I believed it. The facts proved it. I knew it was the truth. I moved naturally back into the magic.

The next time I left the magic, I turned to a close friend, one of the best healers I know, to help me identify the source of my issue. It turned out to be my ancestry/heritage, and the problem originated with my mother's mother. There was no need to identify the generation in which the problem arose. I simply released it from my ancestry/heritage and freed myself from its control. My friend pointed out that if your mother did something painful to you it was because it had been done to her. This one piece of information gives you a new perspective, and helps you understand and forgive her.

As each issue surfaced to be released, I became more loving and empowered. I was led to go back to my ancestry, where the story began. As I let each issue go, I saw it liberating the generations that went before me as well as myself.

These steps have been life-changing for me.

I have moved forward with a new belief system and a new technique. May this book inspire you to do the same.

Love,

Maxine

The Three Steps

THE THREE STEPS TO moving into the magic are very simple.

Step 1

Step 1 – Move into the Womb

The first step is to allow yourself to move back to the womb. This can take just a few seconds. From the womb, you will instantly see everything with a new clarity. You will be alert, awake, energized and uplifted. Most of all, you will recognize the truth when you hear it. You may want to pause here and enjoy the magical space you are in, or you may prefer to move forward to the second step. If you pause, you will know when to move forward because your joy will be gone.

Step 2

Step 2 – The Pact

The second step is to ask God to show you the Pact you made with your mother. You will instantly receive the information you requested. You may want to write it down because within that information is your Pact. You will recognize it because it will feel right. Once you have identified the Pact, release it. You will instantly return to your previous magical state. You may find that the joy, the bliss and the love you feel for others has increased because it is no longer blocked by your Pact. This joy, this bliss, this love is your natural state. It is who you are.

Suggested releasing technique: Relax your body, inhale, and release the Pact to God on the exhale. If you have a different releasing technique you prefer, you can certainly use it.

Step 3

Step 3 – The Bad Message/Good Message

The third step is the Bad Message. If you do not recall when your mother gave you your Bad Message, ask God to show it to you. Then, either write it down in detail, and include your emotional response when it occurred, or speak it out loud. As you do this, be looking for that critical moment when you clearly see that you were not bad, that you did not do anything wrong, that you were, in fact, *good!* Then accept the truth that you were good – and *are* good. This acceptance is truly liberating!

Some people received their Bad Message from their father rather than their mother. If you are one of these people, just substitute father for mother.

The Bad Message

WHILE THERE ARE ALWAYS exceptions to every rule, what I am about to share with you is true for most people. When you were born, the most important person in your life was your mother. She was your all. She provided food, love, security, warmth and all good things. She loved you and, as a result, you loved yourself and were happy. You were an inseparable team. Where she went, you went. Your days consisted of doing what children do: you played. Life was idyllic. It was the proverbial Garden of Eden.

Then one day, between the ages of three and six, while you were playing, you became curious and stepped out on your own without her. You did not do anything wrong, you simply moved forward to explore and expand your world. However, you acted independently, i.e., without your mother, and she lost control over you. This upset her enormously. She may have cried, gotten angry, or turned her back on you. At that moment, her reaction told you that you had done something wrong and that you were therefore bad (for upsetting her by acting independently).

The shock and pain of having inadvertently hurt your mother was traumatic and hypnotic. It was a turning point in your life. You were figurately thrown out of the Garden of Eden, and your life was never the same.

You did not mean to hurt your mother; you were just playing. However, it was too late. From that moment on you accepted that you were bad. You had to get good enough to recapture her love. How did you do this? By curbing your natural curiosity, independence and free spirit, and doing what she wanted. You did this by silently, often subconsciously, making the commitment to obey her and allow her to control you. For some people, this involves holding themselves back; for others, it involves excelling and constantly moving upward and forward. While everyone's commitment to their mother is different, they all involve giving her what she wants in order to get good enough for her. This was your first commitment and set the stage for subsequent commitments. It is in your cells, and unless you have already identified it and let it go, it is still running your life.

You made this commitment to your mother to prove you were good enough to be forgiven. You felt that if she would just forgive you, then you could forgive yourself, and life would be as it was before. If she would just love you the way she did when you were young, you could love yourself. If she would just give you permission to explore, to soar, to be yourself, you would be free to do so. Without her permission, you are locked into trying to get good enough, even if she is no longer living. Without her forgiveness you are controlled by your commitment to her because, in the back of your mind, you are bad (for having upset her). Without her forgiveness, you atone and punish yourself.

Some children, after trying and trying and trying, recognize that they will never be able to do enough to get good enough. Rather than continue to try to prove that they are and give their mother what she wants, they rebel. Their unspoken statement is, "You think I'm bad? Ha! Just watch! I'll show you bad!" Even though they are rebelling against the Bad Message, it is still alive and well, and their commitment to her still runs them. This rebellion continues as they grow up and becomes a pattern that affects every area of their life: work, relationships, career, money, etc.

Some people flip between submission to and rebellion against the Bad Message. Either way, it still controls them.

Your commitment to your mother sets the tone for all subsequent commitments, and creates the different roles you have chosen to play in order to get good enough, such as surrogate mother, martyr, victim, hero, superstar, high achiever, failure, pleaser, avenger, authority, leader, hypochondriac, etc.

The Bad Message marks the end of your idyllic childhood and the beginning of the never-ending, constantly repeating story of your life.

The bottom line is this: the reason you are "bad" is because, unbeknownst to you, you broke your Pact with your mother.

Once you know what your Pact with your mother is, simply release it to God. Let it go. You will know when you are ready to do this because the Pact can feel awful. It was created when you were pre-verbal and felt everything deeply. This is how you will feel when your Pact is activated.

It has been my experience and observation that at this point you can experience exquisite highs and extreme lows until you are able to stay in the magic. The highs are letting you know that you are in the magic, the unified field, where all creation and healing takes place. Some people call this the quantum field, the zero point field, the present, etc. This is where your love, your joy, your bliss can create *instantly*. The lows are the indication that you are being shown something from your Pact with your mother. No matter how it appears, whether it deals with your money, health, emotions, children, etc., if it destroys your joy, it is showing you your Pact with your mother. Remember: everything, *everything,* **everything** begins with your mother and your Pact with her. If your conscious mind cannot see a connection between what is currently upsetting you, simply identify the emotion you are feeling and let it go. Then, ask yourself, "*What does this have to do with my mother?*" Remind yourself that you are God living in an earthly body. This means you are love, truth, beauty, health, wealth, joy, limitless potential, and you have the power to create your life *your* way.

21

If you are experiencing anything less, it's not you; it's your mother. When you see it, let it go.

The next step is to look at the Bad Message you received as a child. You may have done this before. However, now that you have released the Pact, you will see it with the eyes of truth. Look for the critical point in your story which tells you that you were good not bad. This is your turning point. This is your step to freedom. Accept that you are and always have been good.

Then create your life *your* way.

Love,

Maxine

Highlights from True Stories

Bob's Introduction to the Pact

"HELP ME, BOBBY." THIS was the Pact I had with my mother. She was so beautiful.

What's a "Pact"? Something resulting from a spiritual awakening I experienced recently. I believe when you are open to personal growth, you will continually attract more growth, new learnings which enhance the clarity of your purpose and the meaning your life holds for you.

I met a new friend a few years ago. Maxine Taylor was the first licensed astrologer in America. Her reputation is wide. One afternoon during lunch together... "Bob, I'm writing a book. *Secrets from the Womb.* (Her seventh or eighth...she's hard to keep up with!) "Would you like to be a 'lab rat' for me?"

"Hey, why not?" (I had no idea what she was talking about.)

Max explained, "We are all brought to life while in our mother's womb. We share her DNA, her blood, her nervous system for nine months. All of her. We are her. While in the womb, the Pact is born. It's magical. What I'd like to do for you is guide you to uncovering your own Pact with your mother."

"Ok..." "Beautiful, loving, closed, sensitive, sad, *help*." Max stopped me. "Tell me about 'help.'"

As we explored further, I gradually, magically uncovered my Pact with my mother.

She was reaching out to me as I came to life. *"Help me, Bobby."* As I tried to absorb what was going on, I became very emotional. It was as if she was revisiting me at that very moment. My mother was then, still is, a central part of my life. I wrote earlier about our loving relationship. How she had helped me through many of my life struggles. From her support of my athletics at school and college to my bout with mental illness early in my marriage and business career. She was there to *help* me. But so, too, was I born to *help* her? Deal with childhood trauma. Overcome the loss of a child when he was two years old. I needed to be there for her. She reached out to be from her womb. I would be her primary support through it all. That was my Pact. *"Help me, Bobby."*

As I was about to sign off with Max, I slowly turned my head to my left. There, hanging on the wall, was the portrait of a young harlot from many years past. Tattered clothes. Her red hair draped over her face shielding her eyes. Shamed, lost... her sadness radiated as I peered at the picture. I had purchased it in Spain seven years ago. Nancy and I were in an art gallery. She was looking through landscapes and decorative prints. I bought this portrait.

"Why are you buying that, Bob?" Nancy asked. "I don't know. It just hit me."

Suddenly, as I was tearing, my Pact came to me. Mom had called out to me to "help." This picture solidified my feelings. As I thought further, I felt a need to validate my discovery. I called my brother. Shared my experience with him. "Absolutely. You helped her. You made her laugh to tears. You protected her when dad verbally struck out at her. You took her to the hospital when she was admitted for treatment of her alcoholism. Yeah, you really helped her. You were her protector." This was all hard to process. The Pact... the picture... my brother's confirmation. I searched further...

My most successful coaching engagement had been with females. My work with execs had usually focused on releasing their "feminine" energy. Helping them get to their "softer" side. More empathy, better listening, heightened sensitivity. All traits that would enhance their connections with their people. This then returned me to my Pact with mom. I had guided, *helped* numerous females through strife, conflict...even one through divorce. The picture of the harlot connected me with my history of helping females. Just as I had helped my mother for decades.

I'd found an added link to my better knowing me. My coach and I had done extensive work delving into my relationships with both my parents. And the impact both had had on me. But my Pact with mom provided a truly unexpected, new clarity. *"Help me, Bobby."* While furthering my confidence that the path I have chosen has been God's call to me.

"Help me, Bobby." Continue helping others...

Bob's Bad Message

AS A YOUNG BOY I suffered from strabismus...commonly known as crossed eyes. I was extremely self-conscious. My little friends reveled in picking on me. My mother took her shots as well. Not intentional. She gave me my Bad Message. Little did she know the profound impact her Bad Message would have on me.

"What's wrong with you, Bobby?!" A sharp comment regarding childish or bad behavior. But when coupled with the feelings of my crossed eyes? Mom's message cut much deeper than she could ever imagine. This was my mother's Bad Message. Unfortunately, I carried this with me all through high school, college... and to some extent faintly even today.

Today, I'll occasionally get a comment that I'm kinda good looking. Feels each time like a drop of water on a sun heated rock. "Maybe there's not as much wrong with me as I thought."

But then there is the antidote to mom's early assertion. Her Bad Message... "What's wrong with you Bobby?!" It was only last week it happened. Mom's Good Message came to me. Was sent my way.

I've spent decades working with teams, coaching and helping people grow. Now, I'm an extremely "needy" person. Praise, atta boys, anything positive is my rocket fuel. Maybe that cross eyed little boy birthed this in me. No matter.

What resulted? Letters, cards, notes from those I'd helped along my journeys with them all. My oldest daughter Lisa decided these all had to be kept somewhere. As a birthday gift one year she gave me two beautiful mahogany boxes. Today they overflow with the pieces of praise sent me over all the years.

Here's where my mother's Good Message surfaced.

It has taken me days to sort through all the pieces in both mahogany boxes. The other day I came upon a letter written to me by my mom. Her handwriting was unmistakable. Elegant. Classic. As if it just flowed from the tips of her fingers. I picked the letter up and began to read. The occasion was my 50th birthday. My family had flown to Atlanta to surprise me. Mom's letter congratulated me again on my birthday. But then, there followed my Good Message from her. Loving, sensitive. The pride she had in me. All I'd accomplished. Above all, the beautiful family Nancy and I had nurtured. Mom's Good Message could not have been more loving, more supportive of her oldest son. How much she loved me.

The Good Message drowned out the Bad Message. Indeed, there was nothing wrong with me at all. Mom had gone through a lot in her early years as a parent. Too much to cover here. Indeed, her "What's wrong with you, Bobby?!" Bad Message had sprung from the "wrong" in her at the time. Her letter... her Good Message is what I hold onto in my late seventies as her assurance.

"Bobby, you're wonderful. Nothing is wrong with you at all."

Thanks be to God...

Bob's Story

IT'S BEEN SAID, "YOU only fear the unknown." Seeking, venturing into the unknown can be fearful. But sometimes the unknown reaches out and seeks you. You don't find it. It finds you. In unexpected, special ways. Thus was the case yesterday when my dear friend, Maxine Taylor, guided me through a spiritual awakening process that allowed me to uncover something previously unknown to me. Max is writing a book based on the premise that life begins in our mother's womb. Long before we physically enter this earth her blood is our blood. Her DNA is our DNA. Simply, we are her. Much if not all we become in life goes back to the time spent in our mother's womb. It's all about mom.

I wasn't skeptical about this exercise because I love and trust my friend Max. But I was curious when she suggested I serve as one of her "lab rats" for what proved to be an emotional, inspiring growth experience.

I've coached hundreds of people over five decades. As a leader, a business executive and, today, as a Life Coach. I've always focused on "relationship" as the key to the success of most endeavors. Building a career, a business...a marriage. Any time people come together to accomplish something. I call this the "soft stuff." My mission in life, "Helping people grow." It's always been about relationships with me. I've wondered why many times. *Yesterday, with Max, the answer rushed to my consciousness. Like a laser.*

My mother faced a bunch of formidable challenges in her life. Many of them too personal to share here. But I shared these with Max yesterday. Let me give you the bottom line. In my coaching, I've always focused on and most enjoyed coaching women. The many ladies who have come to me with challenges found in females. I always wondered why.

As Max led me yesterday, I realized it all because of my mom. All because of my relationship with my mother. She was a beautiful lady, but she suffered from alcoholism for the first 40 years of my life. She had a difficult, verbally abusive relationship with my father. She had experienced much of the same with her father. I now believe I was conceived in her womb, brought to this life to help her work through these acute, difficult challenges. The message sent to me while in her womb? *"I would be the one who would always be there for her."* As I thought back yesterday, this absolutely was the case. Max's exercise had moved my consciousness from gray to black and white. It was just so clear.

My mother was the first of the many women I've helped, counseled over the years. Helped them overcome their challenges just as I'd done for my mom...since birth. Wow! What a revelation this was! The validation of all this surrounded me. The pictures I had in my office. My remembrances of the many women I'd coached. They all had come to me for help. Just as my mother had come to me...to help her. The exchanges always focused on the "feminine." This was all about the feminine energy that fueled these relationships. I've always felt I had a lot of feminine energy. I could not have worked so successfully with the many women that I did if this wasn't true. Curiously, I realized I was always drawn to men who were sensitive. Men who could feel their feelings. Those who shared their feminine energy with me thus propelling our work together. Another confirmation that mom was the source.

I had a coach of my own for over 20 years. He always referred to "God Goddess", viewing God in the form of a female. As a result, when I picture God today, I have a picture of a female.

I could go on. This was so fascinating. But I awoke this morning at 3am. I had to record in writing the new feelings and emotions that surfaced in me yesterday. I may have more to say, but I've been writing for over two hours. My puppy, and yes, even my bed is calling out to me.

Louise's Story

WHO AM I? WILL someone hear me? Will they actually believe me, accept me for who I am? The good and the bad? Will they hear what I really want? Will they hear what I really need? Will they hear my pain, even when I don't tell them how much it really hurts? Why is it when I talk to people, it's extremely hard to share and open up? And when I *do* open up, I feel I have said too much. I feel I have done something wrong. I feel guilty. Why do I always feel drawn to take care of others? Why do I always take care of everyone, no matter what the consequences are for me? No questions asked, just do what you are supposed to do. Who am I?

It's getting close to the time for my meeting with Maxine. As I look out the window from my home office, I see it's raining. I think to myself, *What will my Pact be with my mother? Will I be able to break this Pact? What will I learn? How will this change me? How will I feel afterwards?*

It's now time to find out, or at least I think it's time. It's now raining really hard. Maxine and I start the process. What is my Pact? The only thing that keeps coming up in my mind is, "You are not supposed to know. You are not supposed to know." Maxine tells me to take my time, but the only thing I can feel is still, "You are not supposed to know." Then all of a sudden, out of nowhere with no warning, my power goes out. I immediately lose my Internet connection with Maxine. I am hoping it's just a quick flicker, and it will be right back on. It's not. The power and Internet are out. My phone then immediately rings. It's my father. I send him to voicemail. We will have to talk later. Right now, I've got to try to get back online with Maxine. I do, however, listen to his voicemail just to make all is okay. His message said he was just checking in with me. I pause for a moment and think to myself, *This is very unusual for him to call to check on me. I am the one who usually calls and checks on him. Plus, he never calls me this late.*

The power and Internet are still out when my husband comes home from the store. I am still waiting to get back online with Maxine. My husband tells me that while he was at the store, out of the blue, for no reason at all, he suddenly got extremely tired. A tiredness that he has never in his life felt before. I tell him about my meeting with Maxine and how she said I could feel very tired, like he is feeling right now. I tell him about how the power and Internet outage interrupted our meeting. He then proceeds to tell me he is so tired he cannot keep his eyes open any longer and he must go lie down.

Still no Internet. I look down at my cell phone. I see I have a missed call from Maxine and now I missed a call from my oldest son, too. Wow, such a short period of time and another family member has either reached out to me or they are feeling unusually tired. Very unusual. *Are my family members unknowingly feeliing me break this Pact?*

I call Maxine back. I still have no Internet, but realize we don't have to wait for my home Internet to come back on. I have my cell phone. We talk a moment and then we get back to our meeting via Zoom using my cell phone.

We continue the session where we left off with the Pact with my mother. I immediately start crying and cannot stop. I tell Maxine," I don't know what this is that I am feeling, but whatever it is, I feel it so greatly."

Maxine asks me to think about this emotion and how I am I feeling about it. I think to myself for a minute and then reply, "I see myself. I am myself. I feel like I don't know what I am doing, and I feel fear. I am afraid. I have never felt afraid and fearful like this before." I am crying. We talk through everything,and she helps me realize that these are my mother's thoughts and feelings. She reminds me that these thoughts and emotions are what I was feeling while I was in my mother's womb. They are hers, not mine.

Maxine continues to ask me some additional questions. I am still crying. We continue to talk through the feelings and thoughts that I am having. Maxine reminds me again, to remember these are not my thoughts, they are my mother's. We continue talking, I finally realize my Pact with my mother. It was: I'll be given life. I will just be there. She is not to worry about me. There is to be no attention on me. I am not to be seen or heard. I am to function on my own. I am to help her care for any other children that may come. I am to be a surrogate mother to them.

I see my mother herself. She is but a child. She is only sixteen years old. She has been given the choice to keep me or have an abortion. She ponders over the decision. There is a fear of pregnancy for her. Part of this fear is being a young pregnant teenager, not knowing what she will even do, or if she is able to do it. She has not yet lived, explored, found out who she is. She has not begun her life yet. This is not her only fear. There is also a fear of pregnancy because she almost died when she was born. There was an RH- incompatibility complication, one which should not have been there because she was supposed to be the first child. She was rushed to another hospital and given a blood transfusion. I feel my mother is scared. She doesn't know what she is doing. She is afraid.

I now can see the Pact clear as day. I understand why certain things happened the way they did, and why I am the way I am. I was molested several times as a very young child by a family member on my mother's side. I see all the thoughts that ran through my mind when I was just a five-year-old little girl. I've played these words over and over in my mind many times through the years. It all now makes sense. I couldn't tell her then because that would have broken the Pact, and I couldn't do that. If I did, I would have been heard and seen, attention would have been put on me. I also felt she wouldn't believe me. I now know why I felt that she would believe the molester over me. This family member was in her life way before me. She had to have loved him more than me and would have believed him over me because, after all, he was in her life before our Pact was made. I am just supposed to be there. So, I stay silent, unseen, unheard, just there.

As we talk more, I now look back and see even more how I kept my end of the Pact. As a child I took care of my siblings, I was the "surrogate mother," and I did so with no hatred. This is what the Pact said I was to do, so I did. So much so, people thought that my sister was my baby. My baby? I was only thirteen. My mother knew she didn't have to worry about me. She also knew that as long as I was there all was good. She could work, play, stay out as long as she wanted to, do whatever she wanted to, and never be home if that's what she wanted. Maxine helped me to see that as a child, I received my love from my siblings. This all makes total sense now.

My Pact extended to my current life. I have four beautiful children, and I became a stay-at-home mom while they were young. (I now see I was, unknowingly, trying to break the Pact.) One of my children is my brother's daughter. She was taken away from my brother and his wife the day she was born because of illegal things that were done during her mother's pregnancy. Back then I sat down and talked with my husband. We decided to adopt her. She was born with many problems. In the middle of the adoption journey, I realized how hard this was really going to be on my children and my husband. I tell my husband, I want to adopt her, but I cannot out of fear for them and their quality of life. However, just as quickly as it came out of my mouth, the Pact returned to me. There is no way I would let her go into foster care. I am her family. I didn't know then, but I now see it plain as day. The Pact was extended and holds true. Once again, I become a surrogate mother.

I go a little deeper. More things are becoming clearer. All my life I've had family members tell me I do not share, I do not open up. I do not talk (although I can talk a lot sometimes, but just a lot about nothing). They say that I illustrate "What happens in my family (i.e. me, my husband, and my children) stays in the family." I start to cry even harder. I just realized this is the Pact. I haven't been able to because I am not supposed to be heard, or seen. I am just supposed to be there. I am to function on my own. I have never in my life been able to share much about anything to anyone without leaving the conversation thinking, *Why do I feel so guilty for sharing? Why did I say too much? Why do I feel I shared too much? Why do I feel raw and exposed when, in reality, I really didn't share much of anything at all?*

Maxine and I now come to the step where I am to release the Pact. There are so many things that are running through my head, my heart, my soul. All of these thoughts consume me, and I am supposed to somehow release them. I wonder to myself how will I ever be able to do this. Maxine now takes me through the steps, the steps that will allow me to be able to release the Pact with my mother. I do as she says, then in my mind's eye, I see a bird flying. It swoops down and around, then off it flies away from me. My tears have stopped. I have goose bumps all over my body. My heart, my chest, my mind feel so much lighter now. WOW! Maxine reminds me that I may feel extremely tired now, and possibly on and off for a little while.

My session with Maxine is now finished. I feel so light in my heart, body and soul. A feeling that is new to me. I smile to myself, I like it. I am already feeling the effects of this broken Pact. I think to myself, *I think my family may be feeling it, too.*

Later that evening, after my session with Maxine, my oldest daughter calls me. It is very unusual for so many calls to come in all at once in the evening, and to come within this small space of time during my session with Maxine. I think to myself again, *Are they all unknowingly feeling what I am feeling?* I'm in awe and very curious now. So, after speaking with my daughter, I decide to text her. I ask her if there was a reason she felt she needed to call me earlier tonight. She said, "Hmmm, nothing really, I guess. Maybe I just needed to talk even if it wasn't about anything." So then, because of how my husband said he felt earlier, I asked my daughter if earlier this evening she felt unusually tired? She responded that earlier in the night before she called me, she felt unusually fine and then suddenly had this wave of tiredness. She continued and said, "I even told my husband, 'Whoa, I just got really tired'." I then give her a quick overview of my meeting with Maxine tonight and told her we would talk more later. I'm now really thinking to myself, *WOW!*

My husband and I decide to make a late dinner together tonight. It's been a long day. As we are preparing dinner, I hear him giggle. I pay no attention at first, then I hear him giggle again. I look at him and say "What?" He giggles again, so I look down at my shirt and ask, "Did I spill something on my shirt?" He smiles at me and says, "No, you're dancing while you are cooking. It's cute." I say, "I am?"

We eat, I take a long bath, and I find myself opening up to my husband. I open up to him in a way I have never done before. I opened up so much that I shared with him some things I have never shared with anyone in my whole life! Tonight, I felt heard. I felt seen. I felt I wasn't just there. After our conversation, I didn't feel guilty for sharing. I didn't feel like I said too much. I didn't feel raw and exposed.

The next day, I am unusually clumsy. I keep spilling things and knocking things over like crazy. All I can do is laugh about it. I also feel a little airheaded, and my brain feels like it is discombobulated, so to speak. It feels like a puzzle has been taken apart and the pieces are trying to be put back together. It's like a patchwork of art in my brain, separated now with small black spaces. My brain is reconfiguring where they go. There is no pain, only happiness.

Later next day, I talk to my daughter again, and ask how she is doing. She tells me, that she and both grandbabies are really tired for some reason today. Has my Pact been broken?

My oldest son comes over for dinner. I wanted to try a new recipe on the grill. My usual intention is to find the recipe and my husband grills it. He always does the grilling and has done so for all of our thirty-three plus years of marriage. I have never felt at ease or okay enough to grill outside, so I never even bothered with it. But today, I found myself standing in front of the grill cooking. At first, I didn't even realize that I was actually doing something that I have never done before until my son comes over to the grill and starts talking with me. We talk and discuss what I am making. He then looks at me and says, "Who are you? Look at you grilling!" I take a step back and think, *Wait! I am grilling.* I didn't even think twice to do it today, but before I would never have even attempted it.

It's now two days after my session with Maxine. My oldest daughter and grandbabies come down to stay a couple of days. We decide to all go to out to dinner. I go over to the restaurant counter for a few minutes to look at something. I come back to the table and they are all staring at me. I look at them and say, "What?" My daughter says, "I was just telling Dad you were over there dancing, and he said you have been dancing a lot lately." I smile. I just feel happy and free.

On the third day, feel a little spacey. I will assume I may feel this way for a minute because my body and brain are fixing themselves. I feel like it's the nerve endings in my brain trying, finding new pathways. Me becoming the TRUE ME. Did my family feel the Pact being broken? Did my family feel my transformation, too? Some may argue, "No they didn't," but I will always wholeheartedly say, "Yes, they did."

My heart, mind, and body feel light and free, no longer weighed down. I'm happy! The little things that used to really bug me or make me mad, don't anymore. I don't know everything, but I *do* know, I will be seen now. I will be heard now. I will not feel guilty anymore for speaking. I will not just be there.

I am ME, and I am okay with that. I am actually *very* okay with that, and all I can say is, "I will ride the wave of release, and my loved ones will feel the wonderful ripple effect of it."

Thank you, Maxine!

~Louise

Claire's Story

I CAN'T REMEMBER A time I didn't feel an obligation to help my mother. As the oldest of four daughters, I was entrusted with responsibility for supporting my mom and dad in raising my younger sisters. I loved my parents very much and wanted to please them. My mom like to cook but wasn't much of a housekeeper, and she was definitely not a morning person. So, my days started early. Changing diapers, fixing school lunches for everyone, babysitting, running errands, organizing tasks like washing dishes, cleaning the house or yard, there wasn't much that wasn't delegated to me to do or organize among my sisters.

I always felt loved. And my mom was my biggest cheerleader, no matter what I did. I was a good student, I had great jobs and successes in the outside world. But in my inner world, I felt an obligation to my mom which I didn't understand fully until I went through the simple steps that helped me understand and release my Pact with her.

My mom lost her first daughter, Rose, in childbirth. Two years later, there was much joy in my birth – I was healthy and wanted. But deep down I always felt the need to compensate for my mother's loss. It came up in different ways – I remember my mom talking about how hard it was after family and friends had given her a beautiful baby shower before she was due to give birth. She felt no joy in baby showers after that. I absorbed that message, vowing not to have a baby shower because I felt it was disrespectful of my mom's loss. I even suggested that my sisters think about that too and two of them agreed with me. So, unknowingly, I carried her grief inside me.

My Pact was to keep the flame alive for my mom's loss of Rose within the family and within my heart – mostly an unspoken memory for everyone else, but an obligation for me that made me a caretaker for my sisters and protector of my mom at a young age and throughout my life. I have carried those fears and misguided lessons for decades. They were reconfirmed deep inside me through other experiences.

Over the years, my parents became more distant from each other. My mom never recovered from the loss of her dad, and then lost one of her closest friends. She drank too much, and she became withdrawn. Before my mom and dad divorced, my mom showed me the love letters she found among my dad's belongings from the woman he was seeing. I became the protector of her secrets and her broken heart.

When I became pregnant, I had several complications that required bed rest during the last trimester. Needless to say, there was no baby shower. After all, there was a curse hanging over me, challenging me to remember my mom's grief. I didn't want anything to happen to my baby.

I lived about 100 miles away from most of my family, including my mom so I wasn't a part of their day to day lives. My mom became chronically ill with cancer for about 10 years. When I got the call from my sister at 1am that mom wasn't expected to live through the night, I rounded up my husband and son and drove to her home. Hearing is the last sense we have before death. So, I told my sister to put the phone next to her ear so that she could listen to my voice and hear me say that I would be there soon. We arrived an hour before my mom passed away.

As my mom struggled with her last breath, I could see blood entering her mouth. I moved closer to her and stood over her, shielding her from the others as she passed away. In my mind and heart, I wanted her to have dignity. Inside, I felt her spirit depart.

Six months later, I was pregnant for the second time. Now in my mid-40s, it was unexpected. It had been a very tough year – not only losing my mom, but two other family members and a close friend had also died. I was unhappy in my work, too. I was content with my husband and son, but I honestly questioned whether I could handle being pregnant again. I felt no joy. I prayed for strength and guidance. I miscarried. My grief had been interrupted, but never healed.

My life moved forward, but I was busy, mostly accepting and content with the day to day of life, but something was missing. I changed jobs, and we relocated for work opportunities. Our son was miserable, missing his friends after the move. I built a new life, adding new friends. But there wasn't much thought to evaluating the impact of so much change in our lives. Then I was in an accident and nearly died. I don't remember anything except leaving the house that morning. Ten days later, I didn't know who I was anymore. But I was grateful to be alive. It was a wakeup call but I wasn't sure who the caller was.

My life totally changed. It took a year to heal and repair my physical wounds. I divorced my husband. I changed jobs and moved with my son to a new city. It was a good move and healing for both my son and me. I had a new life. Outwardly, I checked all the boxes that others see. And I continued to be grateful. But inside, I was still dabbling, seemingly committed to survive but not thrive in my soul.

On to my 60s, I seemed to have one physical ailment after another – physical therapy needed for a frozen shoulder, a bad leg sprain, and for my back after being hit in an auto accident. Gall bladder surgery and assorted other health surprises seemed to mirror the last 10 years of my mother's life as she battled cancer. I survived by checking the boxes. I didn't hear birds singing, watch trees swaying in the breeze, or smell the flowers enough. It was as if I was committed not to surpass my mother.

I've always been a spiritual person, but ran from organized religion in my 20s. Now older, I wanted to examine my faith in God, including the faith I left as a young woman. I discovered that meditation and the prevailing cultural pseudo-wisdom that was largely Godless wasn't enough for me. After more exploration and re-examination, I returned to my faith with a deeper understanding of the need for worship of God as a necessary component of my faith in a higher source. This return has been a part of a new personal journey and revelation for me.

About a year ago, I had an odd but memorable dream. In it I became pregnant again but this time I was 70 years old! Certainly, that had no chance of happening! I thought this might mean I was going through a rebirth of some kind. I focused on additional reexamination of my life and what I wanted for myself in this next chapter.

After learning about the Pact and then understanding how my Pact made in the womb with my mother had influenced my life, I have been able to move forward in a happier and unburdened way, free from obligations to my mom and others. Then I worked on my relationships with other family members, starting with my dad. It was such a revelation! It was as if I were peeling the onion, one layer at a time, yet feeling that it was not a bitter process to heal this way. It helped me understand each family member from THEIR perspective, not just mine. This has been particularly important as it relates to my sisters. Certainly, THEY didn't ask for a third parent among them. They wanted equal status in the family, yet I was given a "greater" role in their eyes.

I continue to work with the process to focus on healing each relationship I have – in my heart and in person where welcomed. I've had clearer recognition of who I am than I ever expected. And I am so grateful to have had the opportunity to help me become a happier person in the process.

Today I am 70 and free to move forward with a new message in my heart. God's love shines on me today. I don't need to keep old messages alive. Once you understand your own barriers and the Pact you created with your mother, you, too, can release it. Let God manage that one for you.

The Pact and simple release process helped me realize that I wasn't obligated to protect anyone else; my job was to create the life of my own dreams – that my life deserves center stage. Peeling the

MAXINE TAYLOR

onion has turned into finally opening up the "Rose"
I am meant to be.

Viv's Story

MY MOM AND I were best friends. She was the type of person you loved the moment you met her. She was so funny you just fell in love with her instantly. We talked every day several times a day. We never fought. Most of our days were filled with witty jokes and laughter. She was my joy. We were happy being creative, sewing, crocheting or crafting our next little creation.

I was shattered when she died suddenly from a heart attack in December of 2019. My world stopped. Months later in 2020, the world stopped turning as a result of the global Covid lockdown . Stay home and stay safe was the message. I was fine hiding away and grieving.

By 2022, Covid restrictions were being lifted more and more. Like all of us, I was finally getting back out in the world when I was rear-ended on my way home while waiting at a signal light. I never saw it coming. I was struck so hard that my car was forced into the car in front of me and I was sandwiched between the two cars. The accident left me broken in half by the seat belt. I had several neck and shoulder injuries, I couldn't walk, and I had a broken pelvis and broken hip. I was feeling really bad. We always said that as long as we had each other everything would be okay. But she was gone, everything was upside down, and nothing was the same. I felt like the world went to shit after she died.

Maxine entered my life right after the car accident. I was really going through the dark night of the soul. I felt so lost and alone. I was right in the middle of recovering and trying to learn to walk again. It didn't seem like the most opportune time, but The Divine works in magical ways. I would soon see that I was in the middle of a breakthrough, not a breakdown.

Where there is a crack, the Light can enter. This was when Maxine entered my life and talked to me about my mother. She asked, "What was your relationship with your mother like when you were growing up?" She also asked, "What's your Pact with your mother?" No one had ever asked me these kind of questions before. Until Maxine there was no one who could even create the space for such conversations, let along take me back as deep as the womb!

What does this have to do with my mother and our relationship growing up?

I went on to explain to Maxine how I felt I had lost my joy, my luster for life when my mom died. That, ironically, my accident happened two days after what would have been my mom's 73rd birthday. I had been robbed of my childhood with my mother growing up. Now I wanted more time with her. It was so hard to let her go.

My mom and I didn't start out as best friends.

When she was pregnant with me, she was devastated to learn that my father had another child the same age as my oldest sister. The last thing she wanted was to have her third child with him, and I knew it. I knew it from her womb that she was so hurt. It was a devastating blow that crushed her. Right in the middle of her pregnancy she was faced with questions like, how would her life and relationship with my father continue after finding out this news? I can only imagine some of the questions and emotions that were plaguing her as her pregnancy progressed. And to make matters worse for her, I was a 10 - month baby. She tried everything to get me out of there. She was sooooo done with being pregnant. After I was born, she didn't want to hold me or interact with me. She didn't even want to look at me.

There was much domestic violence in my childhood home. I was separated from my mom before I was one year old. My parents' relationships ended with my dad beating the crap out of my mom, taking all three of us (their daughters) and leaving her for the babysitter, who is still my step-mom to this day, fifty years later.

My father is a narcissistic bully. It would take me 14 long years to get to my mom. He threatened all of us that if we tried to sneak out to see her or try to contact her that he would take us further away and we would never, ever see her again. I was told lies about her to try and turn me against her. He succeeded in shaming her and convincing my sisters that she was a bad person and a bad mother.

Growing up in my father's house I was shamed by my family for being like my mother. I was told, "You're just like your mother. You act just like her. You look/sound just like her!" Most of the time when I was told this it was not a compliment. I was told that I was bad and not good enough, that I needed to hang up being an artist and get a real career, a real job. As a matter of fact, I was told that that I needed to change everything about myself if I was going to be successful and raise a family.

After getting beaten up and beaten down trying to prove I was good or good enough, I rebelled. Bad? I'll show you bad! I started fighting back and throwing punches when my dad hit me. I got kicked out of junior high school twice. That was the final straw. My father gave up and sent me to my mother's. For the next thirty-five years we would be connected at the hip. We were besties.

When Maxine asked me, "What's your Pact with your mother?" I instantly remembered the promise I'd made in utero to her. It was like I was teleported back to my grandma holding me out to my mother in the delivery room saying, "Oh, babe, just loooook at herrrrr. She is sooooo cuuuuuuute. Loooook!"

And I can remember feeling and saying to my mom while still in utero, "If you give me a chance, I swear you're gonna love me. I'll make you happy. I'll be the best thing you ever had. I'll be your best daughter. I'll be the easiest thing in your life. I'm worth it, I'm good enough! Just give me a chance to prove it!" This was my pleading promise to my mother. Somehow, I knew that I needed that extra month in her womb.

There it was! I saw the promise I made to her. This memory revealed so much. Several things clicked together and I got it! Suddenly I could see this Pact so clearly. The first thing that clicked was that from birth I had been rejected, and that pattern had repeated itself throughout my life.

Next, I saw that I was labeled bad from the time I was in utero. I was a baby from a bad man who did bad things. I realized that no matter what I did or said, the Pact is "I'm bad, and everything about me is bad." I also understood that this was the Bad Message my mother received. Every time I was told, "You're just like your mother," it translated as "You are bad like your mother."

But here's the real truth about me. I have more talents than one human should be so lucky to have. I raised three kids as a single mom and successful artist. My whole life I've worked and been around famous people, and have celebrity friends. I worked as a teacher at Apple for over ten years. Total high tech, high performance, mastermind genius lifestyle. I have lived the life that most people dream of living. At an early age I chose to follow my creativity, my dream, my passion instead of being bullied into being someone I'm not. I released the Bad Message that I'm not good enough. It's simply not true. I am good, and I've always been good.

This has been one of the most enlightening experiences in my life. Releasing the Pact has continued to liberate me. I see things so differently now. I was able to see that as long as I held the promise to my mom, I would never be promised to myself. I see that it was always us and we, never just me. I had kept the promise to my mother. Now what? I was stuck until Maxine helped me go all the way back and see the promise. In that moment I was freed in the best possible way.

Since then, numerous exciting things have happened. I started my own LLC, bought a franchise, took back my health, reversed my diabetes, lost over 50 pounds, and so much more. Releasing the Pact has totally transformed my life in countless way, and this is just the beginning.

I am forever grateful for you, Maxine. You are on a whole other level with this teaching. Your wisdom and guidance take us to the next level! It helps us uncover the old promises, commitments, and programming, and move back into the magic.

Callie's Story

WHEN I WAS BORN, I was loved and wanted. That ended when my younger brother was born. I was almost 4 years old, and life as I knew it was over. Any happiness I'd had was replaced with sadness and hopelessness.

My brother required and demanded my mother's full attention, not only as a child, but as an adult as well. He knew how to manipulate my mother, and if he didn't get his way, he would pitch a fit – publicly, if necessary. This was extremely embarrassing to my mother who didn't want the neighbors to know there was anything wrong with our family. She put my brother first and expected me to do the same. I refused.

Instead, I turned to my father and made him the center of my life. He was a serious, unhappy person. My mother once said to me, "Someday Daddy will be happy, then we can all be happy." From that moment on, I took it upon myself to make my father happy so we could all be happy. It never happened.

My father was critical of everyone and everything, and expected perfection from me. When I was a teenager he said, "I expect you to be perfect. It's only when you're not that you'll hear from me." This terrified me. I didn't know why until just recently when I moved back to the womb and got my Pact with my mother.

I had always felt that my family would be happier if I were not there. I didn't know why, but I felt totally unwanted after my brother was born. My Pact with my mother explained it all. It was, "If you'll just let me live, I'll be the perfect child." Wow! What a revelation! Being perfect for my mother included putting her and my brother first, protecting her reputation, keeping the family secrets, being a surrogate mother to my brother, asking her permission before doing anything, and basically being her servant.

But what about the "If you'll just let me live..." part? The Pact explained that, too. When I was in my 30s, my mother confided in me that when she and my father were engaged, shortly before their wedding, she had gotten pregnant. In order to avoid embarrassment from their respective families, they decided that she would have an abortion. Combine my Pact with my father's expectation that I should be perfect, and I understood my terror of making a mistake: a mistake = death. Wow! What a revelation! What a liberation!

Then it was time to look at my Bad Message.

When I was approximately 3-4 years old, my mother would walk me to a local playground, which was a full city block from our house. I loved going to the playground. Getting there involved crossing a busy city street, so I learned that we step off the curb and cross the street when the light is green, and we stop and wait when the light is red.

One sunny morning, my mother was sitting with the other mothers on benches on the side of the apartment building where we all lived. They were busily talking, laughing and having a good time. I was at the front of the building within earshot of them. I wanted to go to the playground, but that was unlikely since my mother was enjoying herself. So, being an obedient child, I called to her and said I was going to the playground. She turned toward me, waved, and said "OK." So, off I went to the

69

playground. When I got to the stop light, I waited till it was green, crossed the street, and played on the swings. I didn't realize how much time had passed and that I was the only one left in the playground when I saw my father walking toward me. He was supposed to be at work. What was he doing here? He took my hand and walked me home. On the way, he gently asked me how I'd gotten to the playground by myself, so I told him step by step.

When we arrived home, all the neighbors were out in the street surrounding my mother. I could see from her tears and swollen eyes that she had been crying, and I wondered why. She took one look at me and, instead of running over and hugging me, she shot me a look of pure hatred and anger. I was shocked! What had I done wrong? All I knew was that I had hurt my mommy and, for the first time in my life, I was bad. For the rest of her life, I did everything I could to get good enough so she would forgive me, but it never happened. In hindsight I realized that what I had done when I stepped out on my own was to break the Pact with her, which was inexcusable.

Last week, I replayed the Bad Message once again, only this time, because I had released my Pact, I saw it clearly. I saw the pivotal step that showed me I was GOOD, not BAD! It was so simple:

Before heading off to the playground, I called out to my mother to let her know where I was going and to get her permission. I didn't break the Pact! I asked her permission, which was one of her rules. It was *she* who didn't take her responsibility to get clarity on what I was saying. I had been good all along! What freedom!

Beth's Story

MY PACT WITH MY mother was to protect her and us kids from our dad's volatile, unpredictable, angry outbursts and threats of violence. We were to behave, be quiet and "tamp it down." We would do anything for our mother. We can know the truth but not speak of it.

I have long seen my mother as a victim of her circumstances in the era in which she was born and raised, and of the expectations of her as a woman and "a lady." As an adult, I've felt a deep sadness for her because she could not find a way to overcome and confront these barriers. I have also felt angry at her for not finding the strength and courage to advocate for herself and for us children, to "call" my dad on his threats and acts of violence, to cover it all up and proceed as if nothing happened. My "M.O." was to flee, to get as far away as I could while not speaking directly to the issues, but to becoming good at keeping secrets, for better or for worse.

Understanding that we had an unspoken pact, I feel a sense of release from that "agreement." It frees her and me (and all four of us children) from having to live within its constraints. I can almost "hear" her now, standing in her power, demanding and commanding respect (even in the face of push-back). I can "hear" her castigating my dad for physically harming us, and threatening to contact the authorities as well as arranging to take us to live with her mother in another city, unless or until he agreed to get help.

In the weeks since my session with Maxine, I have had the sense of digging deeper into my own feelings about what I'd like to do with my time, who I want to spend it with and what kinds of experiences move me. This revelation allowed me to ask myself, on a particular weekend evening, "Okay, what do I really want to do tonight?" Answering myself honestly, I declined an invitation to a sporting event and, instead, took myself to a music and dancing venue. I'm not generally inclined to go to places like that alone, but I did and had a wonderful time. Perhaps that was a "one small step for man; one giant step for humanity" moment. It felt good to a) feel my feelings, b) act on them, and c) not worry about how it would "look."

I also started a list of what kinds of activities I'd like to be involved in with my free time, for example, what organizational involvements. As a result, I found myself leaning toward the arts and arts engagement, rather than sitting in meetings. I need to act on that – sooner rather than later.

Diana's Story

UP UNTIL LETTING GO of the the Pact, I was merely a surrogate of my life. My mother was the true proprietor, and I merely the steward of it, to be steered in whatever direction and purpose she saw fit. Looking back, the only time I recall ever being able to play the role of a child was when she disappeared for a few months, a failed protest against my father's infidelity. During her absence I felt so free, fearless, and unbridled. In retrospect, I was experiencing guiltless acquaintanceships with my own sovereignty. Her non-presence had brought temporary respite from her incessant imposition on me. Ironically, as much as I was liberated by her absence, as soon as she returned, so did my hyper-codependency. I didn't know this then, but this was all part of the Pact: I was to be her comfort human, her protector, her pawn and her weapon, with the stipulation that I could never surpass her.

From a young child up until my early twenties, I couldn't count how many times she had weaponized me against my father and siblings. At some point, I even perceived my father's unfaithfulness toward my mother as infidelity towards me. Her wounds became mine and her crosses to bear, my tribulations to endure.

The beginning of the end of the Pact reached a crescendo one day when my mother and I planned and executed an emotional ambush on my Pisces father. I had architected what I believed to be the perfect plan. I would strategically present my father's transgressions to him. Then he would have no choice but to see the error of his ways, and atone for his wrongdoings. With the encouragement and support of my mother, I believed that nothing could go wrong. Until it all did. The plan had worked too well. My father had finally seen his misdeeds. However, in true escapist Pisces fashion, he immediately sought to run away from them. He demanded that I leave his home immediately, and return to Florida where he and my mom owned a second house. He swore that he would not come home to her until I was no longer there. The manure had truly hit the fan. We had created a huge mess and had no idea how to clean it up. I quickly reported to my mother, my confidante and accomplice. But nothing could have ever prepared me for what ensued: she coolly responded that I had no choice but to get on a plane and leave immediately. I had been betrayed. Abandoned. Discarded. I was alone. I was enraged.

Very soon after I returned to Florida, and did what a Scorpio instinctively does when in insurmountable pain: I threw myself into a hell of my own making to be healed and purified by its fires, and to emerge from the ashes transformed by failure and suffering, and rebirthed through humility and forgiveness. It was the most arduous and grueling seven years I have ever experienced. But I arose from it with newfound wisdom. Of course, I was still worlds away from being perfect. But through these lessons, empathy and acceptance were forged.

Even though many years had passed and I continued to progress towards becoming a better version of myself, there was still work to be done. I had forgiven my parents and accepted them for who they were, but I still occasionally allowed myself to absorb my mother's problems as my own.

When Maxine spoke to me about the Pact, I knew it was a necessary step towards another level of healing. I thankfully accepted her offer and embarked on one of the most life changing processes I have ever endeavored. After having gone through it with her, I immediately felt the life-long burden that I had carried with me finally dissolve. For the first time in my life, I was no longer beholden to my mother. I was finally free. My life was wholly and completely mine. And I knew that I would never go back. As I look back at the tragicomedy that once was my story, I am beyond thankful for the culmination of experiences, as they were precursors that would assist me in both defining the Pact, and finally granting me full emancipation from it. And for that, I will be eternally grateful.

Kristin Michelle Elizabeth

Up until now, I was desperately seeking answers outside of myself. Who am I? Where did I come from? Why am I here, and why does any of this matter? I always felt stuck. Tired. Not feeling good anywhere, like I didn't fit in. I felt like an ocean crashing up against the rocks any time I had to interact. Yet, I've always been someone others seek out. I have a way of understanding people and seeing into their souls within a few eye blinks of meeting them. How could everyone want to be around me when I just wanted to be by myself? "Why am I like this?" was a question I often asked myself. I thought I was cursed.

That was until I started to truly see myself and discover my gifts. With Maxine's help, I recovered the diamond of my true identity. After all, it is true that

I was made under pressure, and I took that pressure with me throughout three decades of my life. I felt it from culture, teachers, peers, brothers, but mostly my mother.

When I was in the womb, I made a pact with her that I would be the perfect angel who saves her, and in return, everyone else. Before I was even born, I felt the pressure of this agreement and feared I wouldn't have enough to survive once I got out. These fears stayed with me my entire life.

Until recently, I never learned how to fill up my own cup. I was always overextending myself to others to the point of my own detriment. In my twenties, I became a workaholic, and alcoholic, and a woman who overtook ADHD medications and antidepressants.

On the outside looking in, it looked like I was doing wonderfully. I made a life for myself in Los Angeles with a pretty stellar career in technology. I was constantly leveling up. But what no one knew was that I was running on empty. My energy levels and bank account were always low, and I felt so misunderstood and alone. I was making over six figures for years, yet, I felt broke. I felt broken.

Since I became conscious of the Pact, I broke it. I stopped lying to myself. I looked at myself for the first time in the mirror and saw the diamond instead of the pressure. I saw the sparkling dazzle of the star I truly am and fell in love with her. I stepped into my empress energy and learned how to receive life's blessings and all the beauty it has to offer. I recognized that I, too, am a blessing. I saw the patterns everywhere and was able to reprogram them. With that, I discovered my spiritual gifts and witnessed my own clairvoyance. I no longer thought of myself as being cursed, but as someone who came here to help others learn this.

I created boundaries. I traveled to five countries. I began to attract financial abundance because I finally accepted that I was worthy of it. I started to see signs and synchronicities everywhere. I learned to trust them. I fell in love after admitting to myself I do want to start a family, and I do desire commitment. I learned patience and how to be present and receptive.

Toni's Story

BEFORE I HAD a session with Maxine to revisit my life in my mother's womb, my life was unsettled and hectic. I was going from pillar to post and wondering why I was not reaching my goals. Oh, I was not a failure. I hit some goals, maybe a little bit short of the whole enchilada. I never felt like I had the magic touch. If I made $100,000, I worked for every dollar. It never just came; I was never able to sit back and let it roll in. That meant that 24/7 I was thinking about my business, meditating, writing, affirming my success, and visualizing. My natal chart showed success, but where was it? How much more did I have to do?

I took Maxine's **Take Back Your Life** and **Take Back Your Money/Business Sessions.** This changed me and my business. I learned where I was blocking my dreams and goals, and how to change the old thoughts and programs. Life was indeed getting better. Business was improving, I felt more relaxed and enjoyed life. I took time off from work, even enjoyed a few vacations with my husband. Life was good, business was better than good, and my husband and I were taking more time to golf! It doesn't get better than this, right?

Then life changed. My husband of 48 years passed. I couldn't put one foot in front of the other. I couldn't even take a deep breath. All I wanted to do was sell my business, sell our house and run far way. I talked to Maxine during this dark time. She helped me understand that what I was feeling was understandable and would get better. The first year was very hard, dark and painful. But the raw pain left and allowed me to think more clearly and know that I was going to be okay, maybe even better than okay.

In a conversation with Maxine, she mentioned that I might benefit from a session in which I went back to when I was in my mother's womb where I received the Pact that runs my life. I was all in, and a date was set.

At the time we'd set, we met on Zoom. Maxine encouraged me to simply relax. Once I relaxed, I could feel myself in the womb. Maxine directed me to listen and feel. Once settled in, I could feel the love from my mom, but I could also feel some disappointment. My parents already had one child, and she was 4 months old!

The message I received from my mother was: DELAY. This was my Pact with her. My mom had to delay her career. When she returned to work, she had 2 children, a newborn and a one-year-old.

So, what did the message "delay" mean for me? I learned to delay success, happiness and anything I really wanted. In order to be the good daughter and make her happy, I would also delay my life, my success, and my happiness. I did whatever it took to please her. If I said I wanted to do something or be something, she would say, "You can't do that," or "You're going to need a lot of luck to do that." I always achieved my goal, but it was delayed or fell short of complete success. So, I pleased my mother and was able to achieve some of my goals.

As I reviewed my life, I saw very clearly how I had delayed my real success. I was successful by most people's standards, but not by my own. I wanted more on some level, but did not work for the big prize. Instead, I learned to be satisfied. It's depressing to see and feel the time I wasted, the opportunities I did not take out of fear of breaking my Pact with my mother to delay. I will tell you it took a while to settle into this new knowledge. I reviewed my life, my business, all of it. I saw how I stopped myself, how I was okay just to have the bills paid and a little left over. As I grew in personal knowledge of myself, I was able to take back my life and take back my business. I learned I could have more. The classes woke my silent desires. I worked on those programs like it was my job. Business grew beyond my wildest dreams. I applied my new knowledge to my personal life, and I was indeed happy.

Last month I went to a furniture store. I wanted to change my living room around, and walked through the store telling myself I do not have to delay my wishes to change my space around. I purchased a new sofa and recliner. The old me would have said, "I will wait until I see how much money I make this spring, I will wait to see if I have a tax bill, I will wait until I move. Delay, delay, delay. This time I did not delay.

I took the session with Maxine that dealt with eliminating the Bad Message and replacing it with the Good Message. I know my life is changing!

As I mentioned, my Pact was: delay, stay by my side and delay your success, your happiness, your life. But when I was 5, my mother enrolled me in preschool. The year prior, she enrolled my sister, who went the first day and never went back. She wanted to stay home, so she did. When it was my turn, I flew out the front door and never looked back. I loved it from Day One.

Boy, was I a disappointment! I am sure my mother wanted me to stay home just like my sister did, but she enrolled me and said it was okay to go. When I ended up loving it, her disappointment set in and she was both sad and angry that I had left her side. She had already programmed me to delay my success and happiness, and now I was having so much fun every day. Therein lies the source of her disappointment and disapproval.

Saturday afternoon, when I had my Bad Message session with Maxine, she helped me realize that I was never bad, that I did not break my Pact with my mother. My mother was simply untruthful. She said it was okay for me to attend preschool, but it really wasn't. Maybe she wasn't even aware of it, but that's not what this discussion is about. What it is about is that when you carry the Bad Message with you, you end up living it, being it. Maxine helped me release it, and accept that I was good and always had been. And I want to tell you that the insights I have had since then have been so powerful I thought I would explode! The joy I have been feeling is so strong I can feel it in my heart chakra. I have been on Cloud Nine since Saturday.

I hope my story encourages each one of you to sit down, release your Bad Message, accept your Good Message, and live the life you truly want to live. And call Maxine if you need help.

Update from Toni:

Since moving into the womb, letting go of the Pact and getting that I was never bad, I never felt lightning bolts or a light coming out of the sky holding all the answers to the universe. Instead, it was complete peace. I have not a worry in the world. I feel my heart expanding and loving more people with a deeper understanding. I do not have the need to jump on every spinning merry-go-'round I see. Now, don't misunderstand me, I am still very human, with very human problems. My businesses have still not sold, but I know I have divine order in my life and sales will come. My goals are clearly in front of my face, and will work out in divine time.

Misty's Story

WOMB

As I imagined myself back in the womb, I began to feel the strength in my mother's emotions. I was created for the purpose of completing the picture of her perfect family.

I listened for words or phrases to come to mind. In an instant, I felt I was there to protect her. Protect her from what? Then, I allowed my mind to relax as if I were watching a boat slowly move over tranquil water, and suddenly I realized she had set me up for a big job.

PACT

My mother needed her symmetrical, perfect family. She had an older son, and myself, the younger daughter, two years younger, just as she had planned. She had her husband and her house. This meant she could please her mother as she had fit the expectations. When my parents divorced, it was as if I had failed her.

My main role was to believe her, even when I heard her lie, and be quiet to ensure she did not get exposed as a liar. She lied all the time. She still does. I was to hate my father because *it was his fault, not hers.* I failed her even more by continuing to be Daddy's little girl.

She needed me to be like an obedient dog to ensure she was viewed as the perfect mother. The perfect mother to her would prove to be a direct reflection of how her mother raised her children. If I wanted or needed her when nobody else was there, she had no time for me and I'd be sent away. However, if others were around, she had the opportunity to *show* the world that she was perfect. She was raised to believe that disciplining your children created good, obedient adults.

Family gatherings, school concerts, sports games, and adventuring with other families were all meant to display her perfection. It's as if she and her sister were playing a game for their mother. Who could do a better job parenting? Better said, *whose children were more obedient and in line?*

Releasing the Pact took its time. It felt as if a layer of skin was shed from my entire body. Completely removed. I felt a quick punch to my belly and I laughed as I thought, *Gut punch me all you want, you're leaving!*

I began feeling goosebumps cover me like a blanket, so strongly as if they were regenerating and replenishing my skin to form a new layer of skin that is only mine. I felt so light and young! It reminded me of when I was on a basketball team, practicing every day and in the best shape of my life. Only clearer and free of cluttered, used energy.

Everything became hilarious! I found my joy! Buried underneath what once was *her* energy that no longer would be welcomed in my life. I thought, *Wow, there's still another step to this process. How could I feel any better? Incredible!*

THE BAD MESSAGE

One day, when I was about three years old, my mother and I had gone to the grocery store. She always said no when I asked for anything and I wanted this pack of gum so badly because it was so pretty! The packaging was striped and colorful, so it called to me. I asked her for it, and of course, she said,

"No." *Well,* I thought, *she's not paying any attention to me, I'll take it. She'll never know.*

Being only three, I opened the gum once we got into the car thinking I was free and clear. She saw me do it, spanked me and pulled me by the arm back into the store so I could give it back to the clerk. Publicly humiliated and ashamed as I was so bad to not have listened to her when she told me no, she proudly stated that her bad child stole this and will be returning it now to teach her a lesson. The lesson was to never go against what she said, although the lesson should have been that stealing was wrong. Either way, she told me, the clerk, and the rest of the family later that day, that I had been bad. By disciplining and hurting me, I'd learn to never disobey her again.

In truth, she was exposed. She felt her motherhood was threatened because her perfect child acted erratically. I then had to hear her phone call to her mother as soon as we arrived home, stating the incident and how she reprimanded me in front of everyone as if she were proud of herself. It's as if she was grateful for the chance to prove her excellence as a *good mom.*

I felt rejuvenated after releasing the message that I was bad and meant to be her scapegoat! Feeling my energy clearing and cleansing my whole being, I was fully aware that I was restored. All of my cells were dancing with joy. Throughout the day, the tingling feeling stayed and my sacral chakra took the most work. Into the night, the buzzing feeling of love was covering my body, especially through my sacral chakra where relationship energy is stored.

I felt clean! Dirty, old energy was being lifted out of my body and I saw so clearly that I was now free. What a relief!

This was the most healing and rewarding experience, and I am so grateful to be who I am, once again.

Rose's Story

I'M ROSE. I'VE RECENTLY learned that I have been stuck in a loop of the Pact I made with my mother in the womb. Sounds like a run on sentence. It is the way I've been living my life. Stuck on a hamster wheel.

Doing the practice of returning to the womb and discovering what's been holding me back has been enlightening. I've told myself about these things for years, but it never resonated until I took the steps. Going back to the womb of my mother to realize that's where it all began blows me away. I learned that that's where the message/Pact (*Never make mom angry!)*was made.

While sitting in the image of being in utero again, many messages flooded my mind: *Be good. Don't get her angry. She doesn't want another girl. Be a boy. Don't speak. Do things for her. Keep her company. Make her happy. Stay out of her way. Don't ask anything of her.*

She has no time for you. Give away yourself to others in order to be loved. Be invisible, silent, and ask for nothing. Don't do anything to take the attention off her.

I could sense her prayers: *Please be a boy this time. I don't want another girl. I don't want to have to get pregnant again. This is my fourth child.* She even told me that she cried when I was born, not out of joy, but because I was another girl. This Pact enveloped my life. *Be what mom wants me to be. Be good enough.* As a child my mother would tell me, "Sometimes I love you, and sometimes I don't." Frequently, every time I opened my mouth I was slapped. I've often said that at least that way they knew I was there. My mom had no patience with young children, and being the fourth daughter followed by my brother, the Prince, I had to make a lot of noise to be heard. So, I did. I gave up trying to be good enough and please her. I was the rebel of the family, often getting into trouble just to get attention. I was told, "Children are to be seen and not heard," from my father. He was an alcoholic and not very involved in my life.

Who cares about Rose? I have acted out and behaved in ways to get attention from my mother. I felt like I had to shut down my feelings in order to let others have what they needed. During this process of returning to the womb I felt that numbness again. *Shut off all feelings. Don't ask for anything from anyone. You don't deserve anything. No special attention for you. You're not good enough.* This was reenforced when I returned to the womb to hear the Bad Message.

I remembered a time when my mom and I were going food shopping. I was younger than ten, but I'm not sure how old I was. She didn't drive, so we walked to the store. She dropped me off at the library next door, by myself, and told me to stay there. She left me and went shopping. After a time, I realized I was alone and had gone through the books that where there. I looked around and didn't know where she was, so I decided to go home. I knew the way home and started to walk. On the way, a man yelled to me from across the street. I looked over and he had exposed himself to me. I turned my head and kept moving. At a faster pace of course. I got home fine and when my mom came in, she let me have it. She screamed at me for leaving the library and walking home alone. I never told her about the man who flashed me. I was too scared to talk or move. I didn't realize I had done anything wrong. My mom was wrong, and she probably knew it. That's why I got yelled at for doing the wrong things, not for her abandoning me in the library alone. It makes me feel so unloved and uncared for by her. I wasn't good enough to be taken care of. I was of no value to her or anyone.

Although I had this flood of emotions during my Pact session, much of the pain and memories flooded my mind days later. I had a nightmare where I woke myself up because I was screaming in pain from the dream. I was fighting with my daughter in the dream because she wouldn't listen to me. I was trying to tell her about the things I didn't do and that I had no control over things that had happened in the past. I was so upset because she wouldn't listen to me. She kept walking away, shaking her head, saying, "I don't care. I don't want to hear it." I felt that night that the roles had reversed, and I was playing out the roles with my daughter. It was really about my feelings towards my mother. I felt at that point all I ever wanted from my mother was her love. I have chased after people so many times trying to do everything right so that I would have their approval. In actuality, I was always looking for my mother's approval, love and attention. The message I got from the dream was, *I just want to be loved. I just want to be wanted. I just want someone to think enough of me to want me and love me unconditionally.*

When I woke up from that dream, I wrote these things down so I would remember how I felt. Reading it the next, day I saw how many times I wrote, *I'm in so much pain. It hurts so bad. I am worthy. I am lovable. I tried to do the right thing.* I realized, too, that I have been eating my pain, gaining weight and not taking care of myself because I am not worthy. I've been drowning my sorrows. The loss, rejection, and abandonment that I felt was crippling. It hurts so bad. That's why I've wanted to die so many times. The pain has been killing my soul. All my life I have given myself over to others, just to be loved by someone, anyone.

When I released the Pact I made with my mother so long ago, I learned that I am love. I am lovable. I am worthy of giving and receiving love. I accept me.

I felt a powerful white light shining down on me. I know that I am loved by many. I am worthy of receiving love from others. Spirit loves me. My family loves me. My friends love me. I love me. Spirit's love replaces this Pact. I am forever free from this Pact. I know that in her own way my mother loved me to the best of her ability. I am a good person, and I am good enough!!

What's Next?

Past, Future, Present

Now that you have released your Pact with your mother and the lie that you are Bad, you will want to stay in the magic, which is love itself. If you find yourself in a place of sorrow or sadness, you will know that you are in the past. Simply release the past to God, and you will automatically move into the future. You will recognize the future by the impatience you feel. You will replay your plan of action and worry about the outcome. Simply release the future to God, and you will automatically be in the present, the magic. It is normal to continue to see your Pact until you choose to stay in the magic. But now you know how to recognize when you are in the past or the future, and let it go. What if you find yourself in a situation that is so upsetting that you not only lose your joy, but feel lost, confused, depressed or angry? Simply ask yourself, "What does this have to do with my mother?" and you will be shown. Remember: everything starts with her. Just declare, "This is not me; it's my mother," and let it go. Then you will gently, naturally move back into the magic, your natural state.

Life is a Movie

Life is a movie, and the script/story constantly repeats itself wherever we go, whoever we are with. We see the world through our role in the story, and project it onto the screen of our life. The cast of characters can change, even the sex of the characters can change, but the roles they play do not.

For example, if you were the firstborn child and were the center of love and attention until your adorable younger brother was born, at which time he replaced you in the number 1 position, this becomes part of your movie, your story. This pattern will repeat itself time and again until you see it and let it go.

If your authoritative father was cold, unaffectionate, and never told you he loved you, you will attract these qualities in anyone in a position of authority, whether a spouse or a boss, whether a man or a woman. Everyone in your life is showing you your movie.

Once you see it, you can let it go

Now What?

Now that you have released your Pact with your mother and the lie that you are Bad, you will want to stay in the magic, which is love itself. If you find yourself in a place of sorrow or sadness, you will know that you are in the past. Simply release the past to God and you will automatically move into the future. You will recognize the future by the impatience you feel. You will replay your plan of action and worry about the outcome. Simply release the future to God and you will automatically be in the present, the magic. It is normal to continue to see your Pact until you choose to stay in the magic. But now you know how to recognize when you are in the past or the future and let it go.

What if you find yourself in a situation that is so upsetting that you not only lose your joy, but feel lost, confused, depressed or angry?

Simply ask yourself, "What does this have to do with my mother?" and you will be shown. Remember: everything starts with her. Just declare, "This is not me; it's my mother," and let it go. Then you will gently, naturally move back into the magic.

Your Ancestry

Your ancestry/lineage plays a huge part in your life today. Many of the messages you received in utero originated with relatives who are no longer living. It is not necessary to know exactly who the relative is. All you need is the information that the emotion or situation you are dealing with originated with someone from your lineage. By this time, your intuition is stronger than ever, so ask if the origin of your current issue is your ancestry, then let it go. You may find that you are shown more information than you anticipated.

The Power of Acceptance

I cannot emphasize the power of accepting a person exactly as they are, or a situation exactly as it is. When you accept them exactly as they are, you are no longer resisting them or what they have done. This can turn the situation around in an instant. You do not condone the person who upset you, nor do you condone what they did. You simply accept that this is how they are and what they've done. Instantly, you have changed. This gives them the room to change and frees you to change the "script."

You do this step for yourself because you want to be happy.

Char came to see me because she hated her job and, more specifically, her boss. As she described her boss and the way she treated Char, I could see why Char was considering leaving her current job. It sounded like Char's boss just plain mean – and enjoyed it. Char agreed and called her boss a "b---h." So, I told Char to accept that her boss was a "b---h." She did, and immediately relaxed and smiled. Problem solved. Within two weeks, Char's boss left the company. Problem completely solved!

One of my students said, "Acceptance doesn't solve the problem; it eliminates it!"

The Magic

You will notice that the magic is a timeless place of love, joy and instant manifestation. The first time I experienced this I was driving to a friend's house, when I suddenly developed a headache. I felt empowered, and loudly declared, "No! I don't want this headache!" It instantly disappeared. Wow! So, I repeated that with two other physical symptoms that were bothering me and got the same result! Double wow!

On another occasion, when I was teaching a class on Zoom, I mentioned that I wanted to finish in an hour's time, if possible. Fifty minutes into the hour there was a message on my computer screen that my battery was low and needed to be charged. As I announced this to the class, I looked at the plug and realized I had inadvertently dislodged it from the outlet! This event showed me the creative power of words when we are in the magic, i.e., coming from love.

And finally, I was on the way to an arts festival at a large park where parking was at a premium. Finding a spot - any spot, was always a challenge. I said to my friend who was driving that the perfect spot was waiting for us. The vehicle we were in was one of those long Jeep SUVs that require a space large enough for two cars. Sure enough, we turned the corner and there was a huge vacant spot just waiting for us.

You may find that your taste in movies, TV shows, books or music has changed. You will feel more and more loving, so your friendship circle may change. Your taste in clothing or your hair style can change as you continue to express your true self, free from the Pact. Just get clarity on what you want and go for it.

About Maxine

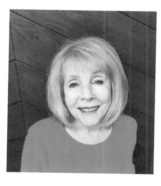

MAXINE TAYLOR IS A true pioneer in the field of astrology. She began her astrological studies in 1966. In 1968, she became America's first licensed astrologer. In 1969, she had a bill introduced into the Georgia General Assembly to legalize astrology in Atlanta, and in 1970, the bill was signed into law by the governor.

Maxine learned how to release our childhood programming, and began sharing her Take Back Your Life method with clients, in private sessions, workshops, and in her book, *Move into the Magic*. She is an ordained nondenominational minister and developed her own healing technique, Star Matrix.

Today, she is once again a true pioneer. This time the subject is personal spiritual growth, which has always been her passion. She has discovered a simple, 3-step method to identify and let go of what blocks us from living in a state of love, joy, and bliss, i.e., the magic, which is our natural state. In *Secrets from the Womb,* she shares these three steps, and includes the true stories of how her method has changed lives.

For a personal session with Maxine, visit her website at MaxineTaylor.com

Made in United States
Troutdale, OR
12/02/2023

15246199R00066